MEDITATION AT WORK

Simple steps to relax and boost your productivity

Written by Véronique Vesiez
Translated by Jessica Foster

Coaching 50MINUTES.com

MEDITATION AT WORK

- **Issue**: as we endlessly extol the virtues of meditation, what can we actually do to practise it at work?
- **Uses**: meditate in your workspace to stop stress at its source and stay focused.
- **Professional context**: stress management, wellbeing at work.
- **FAQs**:
  - What is the difference between relaxation and meditation?
  - What are the different techniques of meditation?
  - How can you be sure that you are meditating 'well'?
  - How does mindfulness meditation develop emotional intelligence?
  - As it is a personal quest, is it not technically impossible to meditate at work?
  - What are the advantages of meditation for an employee?

    "Half an hour's meditation each day is essential, except when you are busy. Then a full hour is needed." (Saint Francis de Sales)

Meditating at work is something that seems unthinkable, even idealistic! At work, we are always being requested to do hundreds of things: a file to finish urgently, dealing with a disagreeable boss, endless meetings, an unexpected speech or conference, etc. For some people, these professional situations exceed what their minds and bodies are capable of coping with: high blood pressure, stress, trouble sleeping or headaches, which can sometimes lead to depression or burnout. So how can we slow down, remain 'zen' in any circumstances and at the same time manage to keep up our efficiency at work?

As far as businesses are concerned, trade unions are taking action in many countries: in France, for example, on 2 July 2008, a national, inter-professional agreement was signed to fight against psychological and social risks and implement collective prevention actions aimed at protecting employees' physical and mental health in the workplace. For their part, employees take individual initiatives to change their pace and give themselves breaks: every way to limit discontent at work is used. But there is still some way to go if we want to regain a calmer and therefore more productive atmosphere within companies.

It is natural that meditation fills the gap by giving us a solution that is original, free and lifesaving. The benefits of meditation, proven by several scientific studies, have led a large number of companies in the United States, Germany and Sweden, for example, to offer meditation in the workplace to their employees who want it. In other countries, managers are increasingly interested in the idea and have started to make it a part of their professional domains.

At work, every moment can become a chance to meditate. Attentively observing what provokes a reaction in us, our emotions and our environment allows us to take a step back and deal with situations in a way that is calmer and better adapted to the events in question. By changing our way of perceiving things, we improve the quality of our vision and relativize our daily lives. Knowing when and how to take a meditative break and/or practising mindfulness at work develops our ability to be aware of what we are experiencing, and to manage our emotions instead of suffering them.

In 50 minutes, discover the benefits of meditation at work and practical advice for restorative breaks.

MEDITATION AT WORK: THE BASICS

STRESS AT WORK

All institutions agree that stress at work is constantly increasing. But where does it come from? According to INRS, the French national research institute, "stress at work arises when someone feels an imbalance between what they are asked to do in a professional setting and the resources they have to meet this demand"[1] (INRS, 2015).

> **Focus**
>
> The Edenred-Ipsos Barometer in 2012 estimated the social cost of stress at work at between two and three billion euros a year, a cost notably linked to absenteeism, turnover, lack of production quality, lack of motivation, etc. According to a 2014 Cegos survey on stress and quality of life at work:
>
> - 53% of employees and 68% of managers regularly suffer from stress at work;
> - Workload, poor organisation, constant changes to the company, a lack of support and isolation are the main causes of stress.

---

1. This extract has been translated by 50Minutes.com.

Business initiatives

In France, an initiative of collective prevention aims to reduce sources of stress in companies by taking direct action on organisation, work conditions, social relationships, etc. According to the Cegos survey in 2014, 59% of human resources directors took actions that year to improve quality of life at work. Depending on the size and activity of the companies, the solutions implemented may differ and include:

- training executives in inclusive management methods;
- adapting work to the employees' abilities and resources;
- clearly defining everyone's roles and responsibilities;
- improving communication of the organisation's strategy;
- giving employees the opportunity to express themselves about things they have noticed are not working;
- facilitating conversations and dialogue between everyone at all levels of the company;
- training staff when new work tools are introduced.

Individual initiatives

To compensate for their companies' lack of initiatives in this area, many employees choose different ways of giving themselves energy:

- adopting new organisational methods;
- evenly spreading their time between their personal and professional lives;
- being able to say no in certain circumstances;
- regularly exercising;

- taking short naps;
- walking or reading during their lunch break;
- hiring a coach.

<u>Did you know?</u>

If you tend to dwell on a criticism or unpleasant comment for hours after receiving it, do not feel bad! This is actually a chemical phenomenon. Criticism triggers the production of cortisol, the stress hormone. Cortisol takes at least 26 hours to leave the body. Compliments, on the other hand, cause us to secrete another hormone, oxytocin, which remains in the bloodstream for around ten minutes.

The longer duration of stress can also be explained by the fact that our 'animal' characteristics mean that we instinctively protect ourselves from external threats.

Despite these collective and individual initiatives, stress remains and persists. Even if we give ourselves a few breaks at work, we tend to deal with subjects and tasks to do immediately, quickly and reactively. This can lead to misunderstandings, mistakes in our decision-making and discrepancies between our way of handling our emotions and communicating with others. Based on a large amount of research, neuroscience now recommends practising meditation at work, as it can have positive effects on our health and wellbeing.

A SOLUTION: MEDITATION

What is meditation?

With its origins in Buddhism, meditation consists of paying attention to a thought (for example, meditating on a philosophical principle with the aim of deeper reflection and understanding) or to oneself (to focus on spiritual identity). While the word 'meditation' includes different methods and philosophies, Buddhism makes a distinction between techniques and objectives:

- Techniques of concentrating on one thing aim to stabilise the mind and calm the individual. The subject of this concentration can be a mantra, breathing, an object, an imaginary image, a sound or a body part, for example.
- Techniques of attention and concentration in the present moment aim to promote understanding ('insight') and wisdom ('vipassana').

Developing our attention and concentration allows us to free ourselves from our internal dialogue, to take a step back and gain lucidity. We are thus more present in what we are doing, more attentive to our bodies, to our aspirations and to others, and we thus become more tolerant and understanding.

By understanding the mechanisms that operate within us and motivate us, we learn to accept ourselves as we really are, with our qualities and our faults. This is the first step towards happiness and greater wisdom.

OVERCOMING PREJUDICES AGAINST MEDITATION

"Meditation does not mean cutting yourself off from the world, but developing a stronger, smarter connection to it." – Christophe André, psychiatrist.

Meditation is not...	Meditation is...
• being religious or self-centred • achieving a result • concentrating • silencing your thoughts • trying to quieten your emotions.	• observing your thoughts • being aware of your reactions • learning to see things as they are • being open to others • seeing things in a fair light • being kind to yourself.

Scientifically proven benefits

Our brains constantly store ideas, process information, make comparisons and recall memories. To save energy, this mental activity is done unconsciously, and so well that most of the time we are actually disconnected from ourselves.

Several neurologists have looked into the impact of meditation on the brain and have deduced, with the help of research and analysis, that the brain changes and models itself based on our experiences, learning and emotions. According to scientific studies, regularly practising meditation can lead to the following changes:

- slower ageing of the cerebral cortex (a thick tissue made up of neurones that surround the brain);
- slight thickening of the left prefrontal cortex (involved in mood, and cognitive and emotional processes), which improves optimism and a feeling of wellbeing;
- slight enlargement of the neurone tissue in the hippo-campus, which helps us to remember things more easily;
- shrinkage of the amygdala, which means less aggression and fear;
- boost to the immune system, which is undoubtedly linked to better stress management.

It is therefore possible, on the condition that it is done regularly, to change the brain with the help of meditation exercises, in exactly the same way as we develop our muscles by exercising! Whatever the type of meditation practised, significant benefits can thus be noticed at different levels.

- On our health:
  - boosted immune system
  - increased energy
  - a reduction in sadness and some addictions
  - slowed ageing process.

Mathieu Ricard, a doctor of cell genetics and a Buddhist monk who is also the Dalai Lama's envoy to France, showed definitively that after three months of meditation, we observe a boosted immune system, a 20-30% increase in antibodies and an increase of stem cells in the blood. Meditation can also contribute to the reduction of cholesterol in the bloodstream and of arterial tension.

- On our behaviour:
  - reduced levels of tension and stress
  - better management of internal conditions, impulses and personal resources
  - reduction in impulsivity, improvement to mood
  - development of self-esteem and empathy
  - improvement in interpersonal communication
  - increased motivation
  - development of compassion and altruism
  - feelings of peace and calm.

According to Antoine Lutz, a French researcher at INSERM in Lyon, "mind-wandering linked to negative emotions, i.e. thinking too much about the past or excessively imagining the future represents around 30-40% of daily mental activity." He then specifies: "When you meditate every day, for 30 to 40 minutes, you cultivate attention, presence and compassion; this has a physiological effect on the brain, on the way in which you regulate your emotions and on the way in which the different networks are activated"[2] (Masson, 2015).

- On our abilities:
  - focused attention
  - improved concentration
  - facilitated learning
  - developed attentiveness
  - faster decision-making
  - activated creativity, and greater independence on

---

2. These extracts have been translated by 50Minutes.com.

tasks.

The businessman Sébastien Henry, who interviewed 60 decision-makers who meditate, explains:

> "Most [managers and decision-makers] started meditating following excess work, burnout or a personal problem (death, divorce). Gradually, the practice was extremely beneficial for them, they feel much less stressed, have better concentration, are more welcoming and more creative, are less likely to be at the centre of a conflict. The work environment is much healthier."[3] (Le Breton, 2014)

GENERAL PRINCIPLES OF MEDITATION

Think about your breathing

Breathing allows us to release whatever is tense, rest what is tired, give energy to what is worn out and be more effective when we get back to work. Being aware of our breathing can therefore be a real attribute for maintaining our energy throughout the day or for getting our strength back after an unpleasant event. Remember that three minutes of conscious breathing are enough to activate the parasympathetic nervous system which creates physical and mental calm.

---

3. This extract has been translated by 50Minutes.com.

Observe yourself

Be attentive to what stirs a reaction in you, your emotions and physical sensations, which can change the way you perceive reality and help you to relativize your daily life. It is a time for calming down and regaining your energy.

---

4. This extract has been translated by 50Minutes.com.

deny that they are there, try to give them a name.
- **I** – Investigate your emotions. Are these emotions normal for you? What thoughts accompany them? Without judgement, become aware of your physical and mental experience.
- **D** – Distance yourself from your emotions. Take a step back: you are not your emotions. They are only a source of information, however precious, about your internal conditions. You can use them to better adapt your behaviour on a daily basis.

Awaken your senses

Take advantage of a food break to awaken your senses. Isolate yourself for about ten minutes, even if only mentally, and call on all your senses to explore a food that you have chosen beforehand (a grape, a piece of chocolate, etc.). Slowly rediscover this food by thinking about its appearance, its texture, its taste, its smell and what you can hear, and fully appreciate this food-centred break!

Adopt mindfulness meditation

To use the definition given by Jon Kabat-Zinn, professor emeritus of the University of Massachusetts Medical School, mindfulness means "paying attention in a particular way: on purpose, in the present moment, and non-judgementally" (Kabat-Zinn, 1994).

By focusing solely on the present moment, we can better accept its requirements. This concentration on the present goes against our usual behaviour, which is influenced by our negative thoughts and expectations, our predictions for the future and our fear of failure. For Édouard Payen, a mindfulness coach, "if we live better in the present moment, concentrating fully on what we do in the moment that we are doing it, we improve the quality of our experiences, our relationship with ourselves and, eventually, our relationship with our colleagues and managers, as we will not be too reactive and will be able to give a more measured response to problems"[5] (Tourmente, 2015).

Whether it is during formal sessions or everyday activities, this practice of awakening lowers our levels of tension and allows us to take a step back from the events. In this approach, various techniques are used:

- meditation on the body and breathing
- exercises on paying attention to internal and external perceptions, bodily sensations, thoughts and emotions
- the illustration of our daily 'autopilot' and the development of our 'being' mode alongside our 'doing' mode
- the recognition of cognitive habits (judgement, evaluation, categorisation or avoidance) that contribute to mental ruminations, and training in acceptance of the present moment.

MBSR

Created by Jon Kabbat-Zinn, the MBSR (Mindfulness Based Stress Reduction) programme is recognised to

---

5. This extract has been translated by 50Minutes.com.

reduce stress and develop an attitude that works with both body and mind. Its users feel less stressed, deal with grief and sadness better, are less likely to develop depression and have more self-esteem and empathy towards others. Studies using magnetic resonance imaging (MRI) have also detected an activation of the zones of the brain involved in happiness, concentration, memory, learning processes, etc. This technique is learned over eight weeks of daily sessions, led by an MBSR instructor, with a weekly session that lasts two and a half hours and personal practice of 20-45 minutes a day.

MEDITATION IN THE WORKPLACE

Have proper breaks

> "Often when people take a break from work, they do not actually have any real downtime: they just do something else. They send a text, make a phone call, check their emails, browse Facebook...these are just different ways of tiring out the brain. But above all, they are not connected to themselves. They connect to their social network, with their social image. But not with their actual self"[6] (André, as cited in Ravier, 2012).

Having proper breaks from work means slowing down your rhythm and using these few moments to revitalise yourself, ground yourself and start again feeling refreshed. It does

---

6. This extract has been translated by 50Minutes.com.

not mean stopping everything, but simply coming back to yourself, calming the rush of your thoughts and being more aware of what is happening within and around us.

Find a quiet corner

Start by finding a place in your work environment where you can be isolated and calm. This can even be in your open plan workspace, sat in front of your desk, as long as you can concentrate on yourself for several minutes in a row. For example, make sure you can put your headphones in and close your eyes without someone coming to ask you questions.

Choose the technique that suits you best

There is nothing like experimenting to figure out what suits you the best: based on your limitations (place, time), find the most suitable form of meditation for you, the one that will not compromise you and which will be able to bring you what you need at the moment you need it.

Denis Machuel, a member of the executive committee of Sodexo, a large French food services company, believes that there are actually two types of practice: "The formal type means dedicating a moment of the day to meditation. It can be 15 minutes or even longer. Then there is informal meditation. This consists of keeping the same quality of presence in our daily lives"[7] (Duport, 2015).

Meditation can be done during a moment of your work day

---

7. This extract has been translated by 50Minutes.com.

especially dedicated to it and can last as long as you wish. In this case, ensure that your conditions are favourable for meditating in peace:

- Go to a calm place;
- Choose a comfortable position;
- Half-close your eyes;
- Choose a centre of focus (breathing, imagined image, repeated word, etc.);
- Be aware of your breathing;
- Let your thoughts come and go;
- Keep your mind focused on your chosen subject.

> "The secret is knowing how to manage your thoughts, not preventing them"[8] (Ricard, no date).

You can also choose to integrate meditation into your daily activities by getting into the habit of truly being present in everything you do, the tasks you carry out and the exchanges you participate in.

Michael Chaskalson, a researcher at the University of Bangor, here gives some practical advice:

- When you arrive at work, regularly give yourself three minutes of mindfulness meditation before starting.
- To re-energise your brain, get away from your screens every 30 minutes and have a stretch.
- Before an important meeting, allow yourself a few minutes of inactivity, silence and calm to re-centre yourself

---

8. This extract has been translated by 50Minutes.com.

on what you have to do.

- Listen to what the other person is telling you, do not judge their suggestions when preparing your responses.
- When you are tense, distracted, worried, worn out or lost, really take the time to calm yourself down and get your energy back, by taking one, five, ten, twenty or even thirty minutes if needed to meditate, with your eyes closed, on what has just happened. Meditate on what you are feeling, which direction you feel you are heading in, and what you are going to decide to do, with the help of mindfulness.

Meditation can also be practised while walking or exercising (doing yoga, tai chi, etc.). This reinforces our energy, stimulates circulation, revives the muscles, facilitates digestion and develops deeper concentration.

You can eventually decide to stop for a moment of "doing almost nothing" before beginning a new activity:

- breathe calmly;
- let your gaze wander;
- observe everything around you in detail;
- listen to the sounds around you.

Practise every day

When meditation is practised on a daily basis, we start to notice the first benefits after two or three weeks. A deeper internal transformation happens after several months of practice. It is essential to practise every day. So make a commitment to yourself! To do this, applications such as Headspace, for example, might help you to vary the exercises, maintain your speed and create some welcome constancy in a highly-charged environment such as the workplace.

TOP TIPS

- Give yourself proper breaks from work! Simply take a moment to slow down, re-energise and start again feeling refreshed.
- To meditate, breathe and pay attention to your breathing. This is the basis of all practices.
- Whether it is time dedicated to meditation, a more meditative approach or the integration of the practice into your everyday life, it is important for you to be completely present in what you are doing, non-judgementally, with curiosity and good intentions.

  "[M]editation helps us to find greater tranquillity, connect to our feelings, find a sense of wholeness, strengthen our relationships, and face our fears" (Salzberg, 2010).

- Practise mindfulness meditation: it helps to develop your emotional intelligence, which allows you to better cope with the demands, pressures and limitations of daily life. You will thus be able to access your own resources more easily and manage different professional situations in a calmer and more suitable way.
- You can practise meditation almost anywhere (on the bus, at work, in a waiting room, at home) and for as long as you want.
- A few minutes a day are enough to take a step back from our daily lives. It is an invitation to leave our comfort zone, and our ways of thinking and behaving.
- For meditation, you do not need training or particular

skills. Nor is it necessary to practise for hours to feel its effects. It is, however, essential to do it regularly.

- You do not have to meditate alone: many books, websites or programmes offer exercises to guide you.
- Be kind to yourself: we have to do what we can with who we are and what we can do at a given moment. There is no such thing as failure, only experience, as neuro-linguistic programming (NLP) reminds us.

FAQS

WHAT IS THE DIFFERENCE BETWEEN RELAXATION AND MEDITATION?

Confusing relaxation and meditation is common. They both lead to a physiological state that promotes physical and emotional health. Nonetheless, they mainly differ with regards to their objective:

- Relaxation aims for a definitive state via unwinding: physical, muscular and emotional relaxation. It can happen following meditation.
- Meditation does not aim to fulfil a particular objective, but consists of being aware of every thought and feeling, and never judging them positively or negatively, but simply observing them. In addition, meditation requires effort that can sometimes be somewhat uncomfortable.

WHAT ARE THE DIFFERENT TECHNIQUES OF MEDITATION?

Among the many techniques, the most well-known meditation practises are the following:

- Mindfulness meditation, which allows us to stabilise our thoughts by deliberately paying attention, non-judgementally, to the present moment and all our surroundings, externally (sounds, for example) and internally (interfering thoughts).
- Buddhist meditation, which is made up of several ap-

proaches, of which the main three are:
  - Zen meditation, which is based on the requirement of the lotus position, which unites the body and the mind;
  - Vipassana meditation, which means 'to see clearly and with deep insight';
  - Tibetan meditation, which is mediation with an altruistic aim.
- Transcendental meditation, considered as a relaxation and personal development technique to reach absolute consciousness, which transcends other levels of consciousness.

HOW CAN YOU BE SURE THAT YOU ARE MEDITATING 'WELL'?

There is no right or wrong way to meditate. It is a personal experience, and it is therefore difficult to make comparisons. Whatever your chosen meditation technique, forget the idea that you can make a mistake or succeed: the key is to take a moment to reconnect to yourself and to your feelings.

HOW DOES MINDFULNESS MEDITATION DEVELOP EMOTIONAL INTELLIGENCE?

By being attentive to the present moment, we can more easily access our resources. The five key skills of emotional intelligence, as defined by Daniel Goleman, American psychologist, which can be developed through mindfulness meditation, are the following:

- **Self-awareness:** being aware of your feelings and using your instinct to inform your decisions. Assessing yourself realistically and having confidence in yourself.
- **Self-control:** managing your emotions so that they enable your work instead of interfering with it. Being conscientious and knowing how to postpone a reward when pursuing an objective. Making a quick recovery from any emotional disturbance.
- **Motivation**: using your desires like a compass that guides you towards your objectives and helps you to take initiatives, optimising your efficiency and persevering despite disappointments and frustration.
- **Empathy**: being capable of adopting someone else's point of view and maintaining good relationships with a wide variety of people.
- **Social skills**: controlling your emotions in your relationships with others, deciphering situations and using these skills to persuade, guide, negotiate, settle differences of opinion, cooperate and motivate teams.

AS IT IS A PERSONAL QUEST, IS IT NOT TECHNICALLY IMPOSSIBLE TO MEDITATE AT WORK?

"We have thought for a long time that we had to leave half of ourselves behind when we cross the threshold of our offices. While meditating means re-centring on ourselves, it is also about being open to external factors. As professionals, we still have emotions. What do we do with them? By letting go of the stories we tell ourselves, we know and recognise our emotions and feelings, which allows us to interact better with others. Meditation gives us a lot of freedom, as when we feel what is happening, we become aware of what is fine and what isn't, and we can act more effectively"[9] (Beryl Marjolin, MBSR instructor, interviewed 26 January 2016).

In this modern view of work, which considers work as more than simply a way of earning money, but another way of feeling fulfilled as a person, to have enriching experiences, to always learn more about oneself and the world, it is clearly not impossible to reconcile meditation and work. This is even more true now as this greater emotional investment into professional life generates stress, which meditation helps to regulate.

WHAT ARE THE ADVANTAGES OF MEDITATION FOR AN EMPLOYEE?

For an employee, meditating can really raise performance.

- Reduced stress: meditation regulates hormones, breathing and cardiac activity, and reduces feelings of stress and anxiety.
- Easier decision-making: by increasing connections between the different parts of the brain and slowing down the emotional centre, meditation gives more time to consider the options in a stressful situation. This allows for better analysis and increases the ability to make good decisions.
- Better empathy: meditation increases the ability to put oneself in another's shoes and understand the role you

---

9. This quote has been translated by 50Minutes.com.

can play in helping them.
- Refined intuition: through meditation, you connect to your body, which gives you access to a large amount of additional information.
- Strengthened innovation: meditation moves your brain away from its familiar routines to create a space in which new ideas can form.

OVER TO YOU

Nothing beats experimenting to find out what suits us best. Here are some exercises suggested by specialists which might inspire you.

ONE MINUTE OF MEDITATION

- Start by isolating yourself in a place where you will not be disturbed.
- Sit comfortably on a chair, with your back straight, legs uncrossed and feet flat on the floor.
- Close your eyes or look down at the ground.
- Now concentrate on your breathing and nothing else. Be aware of what is happening within you every time you inhale and exhale, without trying to change the speed of your breathing.
- If, after a moment, images or thoughts interfere with your concentration – which will certainly be the case – do not give up. Simply refocus your mind on your breathing. Just realising that your mind has wandered and calmly refocusing are the essential basics of mindfulness meditation.
- This short meditation may or may not engender a state of calmness. Whatever you feel, be aware of it and accept it.
- At the end of one minute, reopen your eyes and begin your activities again.

MEDITATION WITH CHOCOLATE

Choose a chocolate bar, whichever one you want, ideally a different chocolate from what you normally eat.

- Choose a calm place where you will not be disturbed.
- Take a piece of chocolate in one of your hands and feel its weight, volume and temperature. Explore its texture by simply applying light pressure between the thumb and index finger.
- Bring the chocolate to near your nose and breathe in its scent – preferably an exercise to do when you don't have a cold!
- Now, look attentively at the chocolate: let your eyes take in its appearance, shadows, reflections, edges and irregularities.
- Place it in your mouth and let it melt on your tongue. Take note of the different flavours and try to swallow it as late as possible, so that you truly feel all the sensations it causes in your mouth.
- If you get distracted, refocus on the present moment: the piece of chocolate melting on your tongue, its texture, its flavours.
- When it has completely melted, swallow it very slowly and consciously. Let it run down your throat.

How do you feel? What did you feel during that experience? Would the chocolate have been better if you had eaten it all in one go, as you normally do?

THE MEDITATION WALK

Choose a flat surface and start walking.

- Be attentive to all the sensations you feel: feel your heel touch the ground, followed by the rest of the foot.
- Walk normally for a moment, then walk backwards, before starting to walk forwards again. Alternate different walking speeds too.
- When you do this, try to feel all the pressure of your feet on the ground, especially when you slow down. A slow movement can allow you to concentrate on other, more subtle sensations.
- Make the most of every step as if you had all the time in the world for it, without an agenda or objective.
- Feel free, if you struggle to fix your concentration, to stop after every step. Close your eyes and become aware of the present moment before continuing.
- You can describe the movements of your feet and legs (for example, "lift foot, remove from ground, bend knee, put heel down") to improve your concentration.

We want to hear from you!
Leave a comment on your online library
and share your favourite books on social media!

FURTHER READING

BIBLIOGRAPHY

- André, C. (2011) *Méditer jour après jour*. Paris: L'Iconoclaste.
- Chaskalson, M. (2011) *The Mindful Workplace*. Chichester: Wiley-Blackwell.
- Cegos. Climat, stress et qualité de vie au travail. Baromètre Cegos 2014. [Online]. [Accessed 14 March 2016]. Available from: <http://www.cegos.fr/solutions/etudes/Pages/climat-stress-qualite-de-vie-au-travail-barometre-cegos.aspx>
- Duport, P. (2015) La méditation se fait une place dans le monde du travail. *France Info*. [Online]. [Accessed 14 March 2016]. Available from: <http://www.franceinfo.fr/emission/s-y-emploie-de-philippeduport/2015-2016/la-meditation-se-fait-une-place-dans-lemonde-du-travail-15-10-2015-14-31>
- Goleman, D. (2005) *Emotional Intelligence: Why It Can Matter More Than IQ*. New York: Bantam Books.
- Henry, S. (2014) *Ces décideurs qui méditent et s'engagent. Un pont entre sagesse et business*. Paris: Dunod.
- INRS. Stress au travail: ce qu'il faut retenir. [Online]. [Accessed 14 March 2016]. Available from: <http://www.inrs.fr/risques/stress/ce-qu-il-faut-retenir.html>
- Kabat-Zinn, J. (1994) *Wherever You Go, There You Are: Mindfulness Meditation in Everyday Life*. New York: Hyperion Books.
- Kabat-Zinn, J. (2008) *Arriving At Your Own Door: 108 lessons in mindfulness*. London: Piatkus.

- Le Breton, M. (2015) Comment la méditation agit-elle sur le cerveau afin de retrouver la pleine conscience ?. *EchoSciences Grenoble.* [Online]. [Accessed 14 March 2016]. Available from: <http://www.echosciences-grenoble.fr/communautes/atout-cerveau/articles/comment-la-meditation-agit-elle-sur-le-cerveau-afin-de-retrouver-la-pleine-conscience>
- Mazoir, F. (2013) Méditer au travail pour concilier sérénité et efficacité. *Modes d'emploi.* [Online]. [Accessed 14 March 2016]. Available from: <http://www.blog-emploi.com/meditation-pleine-conscience-efficacite-travail/>
- Penman, D. and Williams, M. (2011) *Mindfulness: A practical guide to finding peace in a frantic world.* London: Piatkus.
- Ravoir, L. (2012) Vivre en pleine conscience. *Psychologies.* [Online]. [Accessed 14 March 2016]. Available from: <http://www.psychologies.com/Culture/Spiritualites/Meditation/Interviews/Vivre-en-pleine-conscience/2>
- Ricard, M. (no date) Le secret c'est de savoir gérer les pensées, pas de les arrêter. *MatthieuRicard.org.* [Online]. [Accessed 14 March 2016]. Available from: <http://www.matthieuricard.org/medias/matthieu-ricard-le-secret-c-est-de-savoir-gerer-les-pensees-pas-de-les-arreter>
- Salzberg, S. (2011) *Real Happiness: The Power of Meditation.* New York: Workman.
- Tourmente, C. (2015) Méditer sur son lieu de travail pour lutter contre le stress. *Allodocteurs.fr.* [Online]. [Accessed 14 March 2016]. Available from: <http://www.allodocteurs.fr/bien-etre-psycho/relaxation/meditation/mediter-sur-son-lieu-de-travail-pour-lutter-contre-le-

stress_13232.html>

ADDITIONAL SOURCES

- Collard, P. (2014) *The Little Book of Mindfulness: 10 minutes a day to less stress, more peace.* London: Gaia Books.
- Kabat-Zinn, J. (2010) *Letting Everything Become Your Teacher: 100 Lessons in Mindfulness.* New York: Random House.
- The Free Mindfulness Project resources – http://www. freemindfulness.org/download

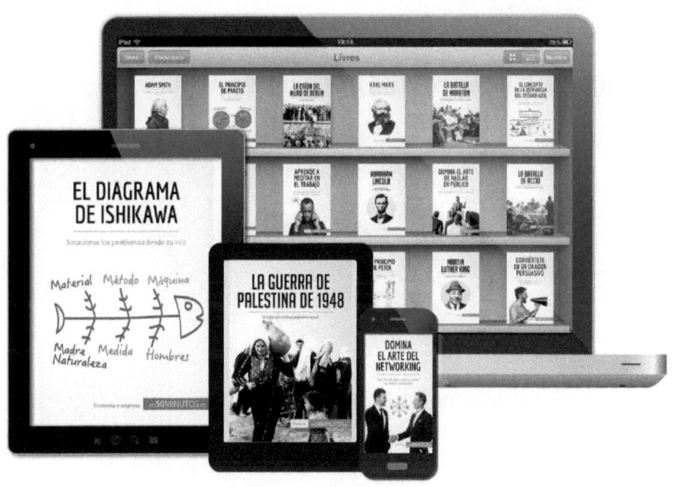

50MINUTES.com
History
Business
Coaching